My Way

My Way

Sandi K. Wilson

Copyright © 2025 by Sandi K. Wilson
Cover Design by SKW Publishing
Cover Artwork by SKW Publishing

ISBN 978-1-7386126-2-8 Paperback
ISBN 978-1-7386126-9-7 E-Book

All rights reserved. No part of this book may be reproduced in any manner whatsoever without written permission, except in the case of brief quotations embodied in critical articles and reviews.

First Printing 2021
Second Printing 2025
© SKW Publishing

CONTENTS

DEDICATION	vii
ACKNOWLEDGEMENTS	ix
DEAR READER	xi

1	The Watch Strap	1
2	Sins of the Father	5
3	The Driveway	12
4	Breathing	16
5	Tuesdays	21
6	Well, Fancy That!	25
7	The Man	28
8	The Old, The New	33
9	Tom and Bruce	36
10	Going Back in Time	39
11	Flat Memories	43
12	Back to the Present	46

13	Where Everybody Knows Your Name	49
14	The Bin	52
15	Three Minutes Fifty-One	55
16	Hands	58
17	The Father	61
18	As Time Goes By…	65
19	The Manager	67
20	Twenty Twenty-Three!	70
21	My Way	73
22	The Final Chapter	76
23	Help!	78
24	Links	82
25	Man of Ivories	83
	About the Author	86

DEDICATION

To my beautiful father Barry,

This book is about you, and in some ways about me.

Together, it was our journey into the unknown.

You taught me a lot, even in your addled state, and the life-long lesson of never giving up on my dreams.

And so, as you cheer me on from the balconies of heaven, I cherish you in my heart and dedicate these meanderings to you.

I love you, Dad.

Sandi xx

ACKNOWLEDGEMENTS

Reflecting on this journey, along with the realness and rawness, there are a few people I would like to mention.

None of this would be possible without the love and support of my husband, Neil. You have been and continue to be a constant treasure in this journey.

Mum and Malcolm, for always allowing me to be open and honest throughout this journey.

Laurie and Tony, without whose blessing, this work wouldn't have been published.

Thanks to my delightful in-laws, Kay and Norm, who have sat tirelessly and shared their own journeys with their folks, and held my hand whilst the tears flowed and the fear was palpable. Your love and support have meant the world to me.

My children - Steph, Jules and Sammy. You've seen your Poppa in all his hues and shades, and yet you delight in him still.

The Staff of Northaven - Dad's home for the last several years. Your support, knowledge, help and care have been incredible. We are forever grateful to you all.

DEAR READER

Welcome to *My Way*, a collection of blog posts written over several years, gathered here as both a tribute and a catharsis. What began as scattered thoughts in the margins of hard days eventually became a lifeline for me. This book is my way of processing the long, raw, and often beautiful journey of walking with my father through Dementia.

In this revised and extended edition, written with the clarity that only time and hindsight can bring, I hope you'll find what I tried to cling to myself: hope. Alongside the brutal honesty and the gut-punch moments, you'll also find laughter, tenderness, and truth. Because while Dementia is cruel and unrelenting, it doesn't erase love. And somehow, between the confusion and the grief, there are still moments of joy. Moments worth remembering.

Thank you for reading.

With love,
Sandi xo

1

The Watch Strap

His urgent phone call hinted at an impending crisis—he was panicked, disoriented, and convinced something terrible had happened to his watch, which he claimed held the key to "remembering things." The desperation in his voice, mingled with confusion and fear, left me no choice but to agree to his visit. When he arrived, he reached for his watch, a timepiece whose broken strap had been a persistent issue he had frequently mentioned. Unfortunately, our location lacked a nearby jeweller capable of fixing it. In an effort to assist, I sketched a map detailing the original purchase location of the watch.

As he fidgeted and grew increasingly agitated, I offered to drive him to the watch retailer soon, though not on that particular day. His memory had become a fragile vessel, unable to retain crucial information such as the place to go or the specifics of his request. In a perplexing twist, he had even sought help from a Super Cheap Auto shop for the broken watch, telling the bemused staff that "they fixed mechanical things, didn't they?" He had wandered in, clutching the timepiece, convinced they might have the tools to restore what he'd lost—not just the strap, but the memory he believed was bound to it, highlighting the extent of his memory lapses. He frequently expressed frustration by physically smacking his head, a harsh self-condemnation for his failing memory.

This disconcerting scene had become all too familiar – a poignant reflection of my father's ongoing battle with Dementia. My once brilliant-minded, fun-loving, and kind-hearted dad was slipping away. Instances like the watch strap dilemma had seamlessly integrated into my routine, underscoring the relentless progression of the disease.

Observing the fear and pain in my Dad's eyes as he grappled with even the simplest of problems or stories was a gut-wrenching experience. You see, my Dad is incomparable, a unique soul who stands apart. Despite the years spent grappling with the various facets of his personality—his stubborn independence, sudden mood swings, offbeat humour, and fiercely protective nature- I have developed a profound admiration for this contemporary unknown savant.

My father, a man of unparalleled uniqueness, had been fighting battles on multiple fronts for years. However, it was becoming increasingly evident that the adversary he faced now was not something he could conquer with sheer willpower and determination. Dementia, with its relentless grip on his memories and cognitive functions, was slowly but surely taking him away from us.

As we navigated through the challenges of his failing memory, the once vibrant and creative mind that had given life to beautiful melodies and heartfelt stories was slipping into the shadows of forgetfulness. It was painful to witness a man who had been such a light and source of inspiration grapple with the fragments of his own recollections.

Despite the hardships, there was a beauty in the moments of clarity that occasionally shone through. In those precious instances, my father's true essence, his kindness, humour, and the unique brilliance that defined him, flickered like a distant star. These moments became treasured fragments, reminders of the incredible person he had been.

The journey through the labyrinth of Dementia was fraught with emotional turbulence—like the time he called me in tears because he couldn't remember how to make his favourite cup of coffee, or when he accused the neighbours of stealing his recycling bin, only to later find it at the back of his unit. Each incident was a painful reminder of how much had changed and how far we had already travelled down this uncertain road. It required a delicate balance of compassion, patience, and acceptance. Every forgotten name, misplaced item, or confused expression etched a bittersweet narrative of a man who had once been a pillar of strength and creativity.

As his caregiver, I found myself adapting to a role I never anticipated. It involved not only attending to his physical needs but also becoming a guardian of his memories, a keeper of the stories that shaped his life. It was an arduous task, yet one filled with moments of profound connection that transcended the limitations imposed by his deteriorating mental state.

In facing the realities of my father's journey with Dementia, I discovered the resilience of love. It was a love that persisted beyond the confines of memory loss, a love that found expression in shared smiles, comforting touches, and the unwavering commitment to preserving the essence of a remarkable individual.

As the chapters of his life unfolded in this uncharted territory of cognitive decline, I clung to the fragments of his true self, determined to honour the legacy of the man who had shaped my world in countless ways.

The journey through Dementia was a painful odyssey—much like that broken watch strap, frayed and useless on its own, yet treasured because it once tethered something valuable. It became a symbol of all we tried to hold together as pieces of him slipped away, but within the heartache, there emerged a poignant celebration of a life well-lived and a love that endured despite the eroding sands of time.

2

Sins of the Father

I had people over for dinner, the table set with candles flickering against the windowpanes and the hum of laughter warming the room, when the phone rang—shrill, insistent, and oddly out of place. The interruption cut through the cosy domestic scene like a blade, foreshadowing the chaos that was about to unfold.

"Sorry to disturb you, Sweetheart, but I was wondering if you could come over first thing tomorrow morning so I can borrow you for five minutes?"
"Sure, Dad, what's up?" Long silence......
"I don't have my car anymore."
"Why not?"
"The Police have taken it."
"Why, Dad?"
"They stopped me and said I was speeding, and they took it, then they brought me home. I've been beaten up by the officer, who was a nasty and violent man. The handcuffs ripped my wrist to shreds."

"Dad, were you arrested?"
"Yes."

I told him I'd come first thing and see what the story was.

I was utterly stunned. My Dad is frail and puffs after checking his mail every day. Why on earth was he arrested? He's a seventy-six-year-old pensioner who lives a very ordinary, if not dull, existence.

I didn't sleep much that night. All sorts of thoughts came flying in and out of my head. So after praying, I got a wee bit of rest, but I was somewhat anxious about what state he would be in.

I wasn't prepared for what met me at the door.

His wounds were real, and they were all over his body—an angry welt where the handcuffs had bitten into his wrist, bruises darkening his arms like ink stains, and a deep gash along his knee that looked jagged and fresh. His wrist was tightly wrapped by the arresting officer and had swelled up to twice its normal size. I carefully cut it off and redressed all his wounds, weeping silently as I did so.

He proceeded to go into the story with all the enthusiasm and drama of an Oracle. He sounded utterly convincing, but for one fact - Dementia has given my Dad a wicked temper, and he no longer has any kind of filter over his mouth.

I rang through to the doctor and got him an immediate appointment. He had to have stitches in his right hand and in his right knee.

Somehow, I whipped up the courage to ring the police later that day, and strangely enough, I got put straight through to the arresting officer. His story and Dad's were poles apart, and somehow I was going to have to find the truth in the middle somewhere.

Mail started to arrive that Dad utterly refused to open—a stack of ominous envelopes accumulating on the kitchen counter like silent witnesses to a life unravelling. The weight of their contents became evident as I coaxed him into opening them, each letter revealing another layer of legal or financial trouble. The more we uncovered, the more I felt the ground shift beneath me. It was as though I had stepped into someone else's nightmare, only to realise it was my own family's reality; and when I managed to get him to open them, we were met with quite a handful of surprises. Dad was fined and due to go to court for 'failure to stop with red and blue lights and siren going.' His refusal to appear could result in a $10,000 fine. Great, what to do now? He was also adamant that we needed to do a Police Complaint against the arresting officer. He had stated that he was met with undue force, thrown to the ground and beaten. Unfortunately, for a frail older man who had no meat on his bones, his injuries looked consistent with this accusation.

Upon reviewing a video that was taken of the car chase, and speaking with the arresting officer, the Police Complaint came to nothing. It turns out Dad had a much more significant part to play; he resisted arrest, swore incessantly at the officer, refused to hand over his car keys and kept yelling at said officer. His car was impounded for a month. His driver's license was revoked for good.

Guess who now became his part-time carer and chief taxi driver—me, juggling my own responsibilities while suddenly plunged into the role of caretaker. I was no longer just a daughter, but a nurse, chauffeur, administrator, and emotional anchor. The daily routine became relentless: driving him to appointments, preparing meals he barely touched, sitting through his angry tirades, and watching the man who once stood tall dissolve before my eyes. I was exhausted—body, mind, and spirit. This unexpected role stretched every part of me, revealing limits I didn't know I had and strength I didn't know I needed, six days a week for months. I became his nurse and took him to his many medical appointments. I became his chief cook and sandwich maker. I took care of his rent and bills and ensured he bought enough food. I would clean his flat while he sat and watched TV. I became tired, stressed, and exhausted. The system we had now entered took a long time to go from the first phone call asking for help to actually receiving the help.

I asked many questions of God and received only one answer; I am able to deal with this. I fight and say I can't, but actually, I could and I did.

I take a lot of deep breaths. I took a step forward and dragged Dad with me, ever moving forward.

Dad's days of freedom and independence were numbered. It wouldn't be long until he would have to go into a home.

His health suffered. His flat, whilst relatively clean and tidy, was never aired, the windows never got opened, and the curtains remained firmly shut. I worried the mould spores would start attacking his lungs. Fortunately, that didn't happen.

Remembering which clothes he had worn and which to put in the wash became a nightmare. Dad slept in his clothes. He wasn't sleeping well and ate very little. His once ample waistline and chubby cheeks melted into a small sixty-four-kilogram frame. My father was wasting away – my beautiful, handsome, vivacious father would all too soon become a memory.

Dad insulted my husband and me at every turn. When he first told us his landlady was 'kicking him out', he had no idea what to do. No idea that he now had to find alternative accommodation, and so it was left up to me. He ended up liking a fully furnished flat in the next Bay along from us. Little did I know how much his presence up here would affect and indeed, change all of us.

My father, in his ultimate wisdom, had pretty much turfed as much of his gear in every concrete rubbish bin along the sprawling Peninsular. I'd hate to think what he managed to get into those receptacles, all I knew was that Dad hadn't bought a council rubbish bag or recycled in years.

From the time he moved up here till the time he was put in a facility, Dad was ever-present and ever-calling. He didn't have a phone in those first few weeks, so he turned up here three times a day. Eventually, the children and I learned to quietly lock the door and hide upstairs, until he walked along our deck, got back into his car and left. I hated doing that, but my sanity was being tested by a demanding, manipulative, repetitive monster hiding in my Dad's body! I guess this started our journey into learning boundaries.

My husband was the one who helped install the phone, the computer, the internet/Wi-Fi, and all things technical. Dad didn't like it, so he would insult hubby at any given time and tell him he was doing everything wrong. Interestingly, it could have been a bonding time, as he once worked for a Telephone company and some of this would have been familiar to him. Dad's Modus Operandi was to then contact my brother, whose "brain worked much better than my husband's!" I'd had enough one day of Dad standing in my home and insulting my husband, who quite frankly didn't have to do a darn thing for this 'feral beast' within the man, and so I made Dad leave – for the first time in my life, I kicked my father out of my home.

I needed to cool off. I was exhausted, and the pressure was getting to me. After a couple of hours, I went around to Dad's place and we made peace with each other. From that day onwards, Dad's attitude towards my husband changed for the better.

Dad's new life up here seemed to carry on for a while, once we got all the things sorted that needed to be. He genuinely seemed to like being so close to the beach, and would often get himself an ice cream, walk across the road and sit at one of the tables, watching all the yachts, boats and children out in the water. I guess it was serendipity finding him a flat (apartment) across from the beach and the Yacht Club.

His days of ringing endlessly and turning up unexpectedly started to calm down, and we all found a new normal to live within. He was still driving around and shopping on his own at this point, and still telling me how "dumb, useless and stupid" I was at every turn.

I was wise enough to know that everything he yells at me is his own heart and thoughts speaking of himself.

Even before Dementia hit, Dad wasn't too involved with us children. He rarely came to his grandchildren's school events, or took too much of an interest in things outside of his immediate world. Dad had chased every dream and done everything he wanted, at the cost of his family. It's no wonder that each of us children, whilst maintaining a good relationship with mum, ended up finding surrogate parents along the way.

The grief that started to envelop me, the tears that started to fall, were not going unnoticed. My husband's parents went through this with his grandparents, and they became an incredible source of strength and knowledge.

As I grappled with the emotional turbulence of this journey, I clung to the hope that, in this new environment, he would find the peace that had eluded him for so long. The challenges remained, but within the pain and uncertainty, a quiet strength blossomed—one that allowed me to navigate the complexities of dementia with grace, resilience, and an enduring love for the man who, despite the tumult, remained my father.

3

The Driveway

My face went pale. I felt sick, as though the world had tilted on its axis. The late afternoon sun, warm just moments before, seemed to dim behind a haze of disbelief. Then the tears started to flow, silent and hot, blurring my vision as a groan escaped my lips, low, guttural, and rising from a place so deep I didn't know it existed. The familiar world around me—the garden, the drive, the chirping birds- suddenly felt unreal, like props on a stage I no longer recognised. And a groan was uttered from my lips that had started deep within my belly.

I couldn't believe what I was hearing.

Then she held me and propped me up so I didn't fall on the driveway.

She was telling me my father was terminal. That his Dementia wasn't just progressing—it was going to kill him. The weight of those words hit me with finality I hadn't expected, even though I thought I'd been bracing for this moment. She told me he was ready for a Care Home now that his judgment was severely impaired already, and he was going to get worse. Then she told me the results from Friday's MRI Scan were in; Dad's Dementia was rapidly growing, and there was a marked increase from the one done over a year ago. He also suffered from Brain Atrophy, a marked decrease in the size of the brain.

There was a lot of news from the Gerontology Nurse that day. A day that changed my life forever. It was a Monday.

My first thought was, how do I tell the boys? The boys are my brothers. Both were grown adults, older than me. But still, I knew those phone calls were going to be heartbreaking. Argh. I also had to ring my daughter in the United Kingdom. There was no one else who would do this, and so the decision was made for me. Lovely.

Nothing can prepare you for hearing the sobs down the end of the phone, nothing. Oh, the curse of time zones and distance, when all you want to do is reach down that line and hug your loved ones at the other end.

By contrast, nothing prepares you for the one who seems to hold it all together. The tears haven't flowed, and the rigidity stays the same. You almost want to slap them with a wet fish and scream, "wake up!" It took a while to realise we all process and grieve in different ways.

Terminal. It conjures up images that are pretty horrid; hospital scenes with emaciated individuals, scarves wrapped around heads, tubes coming out of bodies. Nothing good to look forward to here. And the second image that popped into my head was a gate/terminal at an airport to go through - I could do with that right now.

On average, with the kind of Dementia Dad has, they are given a sentence of around eight years. Dad is about halfway through that now. Interestingly enough, Dad has expressed to me several times that he doesn't want to see his eightieth birthday. I always wondered why.

I had to sit him down and tell him what the nurse had told me. He looked at me and declared, "Well, I do what I want to do and I don't do what I don't want to do. As long as I can get my hair cut tomorrow, I don't give a damn!"

And there you have it. My father doesn't want to know. He wants to keep on living in his flat, but he knows deep down that he can't. He wants to keep up his routine, but that's hard when you are no longer allowed to drive. He wants to keep his world as it is, and yet it is changing at such a fast pace. And I seem to be the one driving him towards this massive change.

Originally, Dad was diagnosed years prior to this by his former doctor. I remember one visit when the doctor gently suggested it might be time to think about home help. Dad scoffed, waved it off with a gruff "I'm not ready for the loony bin yet," and changed the subject. The doctor would often call me privately, urging me to prepare—power of attorney, an updated will, and long-term care plans. But Dad wasn't having a bar of it back then, and neither was I quite ready to confront the reality. Looking back, those calls were like warning bells, but they were easy to ignore when Dad seemed so full of life. It was divine providence indeed that just a few months before Dad's arrest, my brother and I, along with him, went back to his original lawyer and had his will changed, and Power of Attorney sorted out. I had no idea how important this decision was to play in the near future.

The strength and courage that I have been given to do this particular part of Dad's journey has been nothing short of miraculous.

Dad isn't a burden per se; he's actually a bit of a hoot. Like the time he insisted on wearing two different shoes to the chemist because "one was for comfort and the other for speed." Or when he offered a bewildered teenager at the supermarket his expert advice on how to pick a ripe banana, while holding a can of baked beans. These moments make me laugh through the tears.

The things that can be a problem are the medical system and its lack of information. The lack of communication between father and sons. The notion that some stupid doctor is going to give us a timeline when in reality, there is none. It's the little things like now having to turn around and find a care home, one that will meet Dad's needs and be comfortable and without that 'smell' – you know what I'm saying!

Dad's endless stories, which by now are so mixed up and unreal, and yet he is utterly convinced they are true. It's the endless arguments and yelling that transpire when he can't get his way. I almost put him on the side of the road one week after almost causing a car accident.

And so here we are. Yes, here we are indeed.

I'm just remembering a time when Dad rang me with the all-important task of buying bananas!

4

Breathing

I find myself breathing very deeply of late—slow, grounding breaths that seem to remind my body that I'm still here, still standing. It's as though my lungs are trying to create space for everything I've held in: the grief, the exhaustion, the unexpected peace that comes with surrender. These deep breaths have become my way of reclaiming the fragments of myself scattered through months of turmoil. I shudder when I think of what the previous five months have brought to us as a family, and to us as children. But breathing is great. Walking is fantastic. Having my life partially back is a very good thing.

But I miss him.

I miss hearing Dad's loving voice on the phone. He was pretty much always sweet and loving on the other end of the phone.

But now he's in a Secure Dementia Ward.

I had dreaded going there. Whenever he saw me, I was never greeted with a smile or a wave; it was always, "Oh God" or "Oh Jesus". I hate his blaspheming, and I would tell him in an authoritative voice to "cut that out." He would rarely smile, and his demeanour was usually fraught with agitation and anger. I would try to smile and joke with him, trying to bring love and light into his darkness, but he was further away from me at this point than he had ever been. He assaulted me one time, but I turned on him and said very loudly, drawing a firm line I never thought I'd have to make with my own father. My heart was pounding—not just from fear, but from the sorrow of confronting someone I loved in that way. In that moment, I wasn't just protecting myself; I was protecting the fragile bond we still had. "If you ever do that again, I will not take you back to your favourite café!" To this day, Dad has not been that aggressive with me again. Others, yes, but me, no.

I had to stop visiting for a couple of weeks after demanding they change his medication.

It worked. He became my kind father again, well, sort of.

I had to learn some things and make other things a priority in my life now that Dad was in care. It was a hard journey at times, but I had to learn to let go. I'd done everything I could; there would be ebbs and flows, but I, too, had to learn to live differently now.

I literally had his whole world in my garage, and that was now my focus. Emptying it all out so I could actually park my car in there again. At times, I would bring Dad up here, and he would show me what he wanted to keep and what could go. In fact, most things he told me to take to the dump or put in the rubbish, which I mostly did.

There's the desk from my early childhood days, a silent witness to so much of our family's history and the shifting tides of my relationship with Dad. Sitting at that desk now feels like touching a piece of him; before Dementia, before the outbursts, before the distance. It reminds me that there were good days, creative days, shared moments around something as ordinary as furniture. That desk, once a place of play and imagination, now anchors me to the tenderness that still lingers beneath the pain. I lifted off the hardboard that Dad had put on the surface to cover the graffiti. Underneath were etched into the wood, scribblings and scrawl from my eldest brother, with all his favourite bands glaring back at me. I used to love that desk. We've all sat there and done some kind of work, whether homework or being creative. Making model aeroplanes, such as my middle brother did, or me sitting there on mum's old typewriter, practising away. Yes, it's great to have that desk back, but where to put it, nobody knows?

The photos are fantastic. So many memories of wonderful grandparents, relatives, family friends, holidays, and awesome celebrations. Those have stayed here, much laughter and stories lie with those candid shots.

I am grateful for today. While there is still a sense of ultimate responsibility for Dad's welfare, I am so glad that he is in a place which has seen him flourish in a sense, and regain some lost weight. He enjoys it when a local pianist comes in once or twice a week with his keyboard and sings away. He loves playing games and being read to, but his reading skills are no longer there. He gets on with most of the residents, but gosh, he does love it when we arrive to take him out.

I am also saddened. I am still left knowing things about Dad that I wish I never knew—things tucked into drawers, buried in boxes, scribbled in forgotten journals. Hints of decisions and desires that jarred against the man I thought I knew. Each discovery felt like a quiet betrayal, not just of my trust, but of the story I had told myself about who he was.

This all came about when I was single-handedly responsible for clearing out his flat, sorting through what to keep and throw, cleaning the whole dwelling, and dealing with all his finances. Within his belongings were things that told me a story of years gone by that I had never known. I made sure that certain things were returned or destroyed.

In the aftermath of these revelations, my role as a daughter has been reshaped, burdened by the weight of secrets uncovered and responsibilities shouldered. The process of sifting through Dad's past, uncovering hidden chapters, and managing the intricacies of his life has left me grappling with a blend of emotions—love, sadness, and a persistent sense of duty.

The garage, once a repository of memories and forgotten artefacts, has become both a physical and metaphorical battleground. Amidst the tangible remnants of Dad's life, I grapple with the intangible—the stories he chose not to share, and the burdens he carried in silence. It's a delicate dance of understanding and acceptance, acknowledging that every person carries within them layers of complexity, hidden from the prying eyes of loved ones. In sorting through the mess, I'm slowly piecing together what it means to grieve someone who is still alive, and to find peace not just in what's remembered, but in what's released. The garage, once a repository of memories and forgotten artefacts, has become both a physical and metaphorical battleground. Amidst the tangible remnants of Dad's life, I grapple with the intangible—the stories he chose not to share, and the burdens he carried in silence. It's a delicate dance of understanding and acceptance, acknowledging that every person carries within them layers of complexity, hidden from the prying eyes of loved ones.

5

Tuesdays

I walked into the Social Welfare office one morning, and the lady behind the counter recognised me from all the visits I had taken there with Dad. To my shock, she sat there and started to tell me what a great job I had done looking after Dad. Her words caught me completely off guard. For a moment, I didn't know whether to cry, laugh, or deflect the compliment altogether. I wasn't used to being praised for something that had felt more like survival than success. But in that quiet, awkward moment, I felt seen, like maybe I hadn't entirely failed after all. And handling him when he was at his worst. Unfortunately, she had seen Dad get all aggressive, but she had the strategies in place to get him sorted – mine were just basic instincts.

So after this particular visit, I took some time to reflect on what a year it had been for the family, for Dad and for myself.

I've learnt a lot along the way—the right way of doing things, like giving him space when he's overwhelmed and sticking to a predictable routine; and the wrong way, like trying to reason with him when he's in a heightened state or forgetting to bring the Lemon Coconut Slice. Each success and mistake has shaped the way I approach not only his care, but also how I communicate and connect with him, and the way that is best for all concerned.

I remember writing previously about the pain of missing Dad, of not hearing his voice down the phone or being able to pop round and see him regularly. Over time, it had gotten better, but there were days it was still difficult.

We've gone from being greeted with, "Oh God, it's you" to "it's so wonderful to see you, darling. Look, everybody, it's my sister!" Then the realisation that it's actually me, his daughter and then he proclaims, "It's my daughter, isn't she beautiful?" Either way, it's just lovely to be greeted with such warmth and care.

Dad is certainly a creature of habit and schedule. If you change anything even slightly, he notices. I remember once, I parked in a different spot than usual outside the café, and he refused to get out of the car until I explained why. "That's not where we park," he said, arms crossed like a stubborn schoolboy. The familiar rhythm of his routine is his anchor—any disruption feels like a storm.. If you change anything even slightly, he knows and he lets you know. I've learned this past year that he doesn't like a lot of noise, he cannot cope with too many people at once, and he really loves his Lemon Coconut Slice from the local café. I've also come to see quite a massive change in the way he relates to people now.

Don't get me wrong, he still has utterly embarrassing moments where we have to tell him to "shush", and promptly apologise on his behalf. But in general, he genuinely seems interested in everything you tell him. When I told him today that I had just finished writing a book and that I'd submitted it to a Publisher, his eyes popped wide and his response was, "Well, fancy that!" That is massive compared to the rolling of eyes that welcomed me just a few short months beforehand.

Tuesdays were the day that I would go down and pick up Dad and take him to his favourite coffee shop, a nice café on the corner of the street; the hum of the espresso machine, and the smell of cinnamon and warm scones hanging in the air. The same people always served us, greeting Dad by name and remembering his usual order with a wink. The window seats were his favourite; he liked to watch people walk by and comment on their outfits or whether they looked like they were in a hurry. He also loved seeing the pigeons up on the roof of the building across the street. These small rituals gave him something to look forward to, and me too, if I'm honest. The familiarity of it all helped us both settle into a rhythm we didn't know we needed. The café was conveniently located right across from the ANZ bank, a spot that would often trigger Dad's enthusiastic conversations about money and his dreams of returning to Australia. I kept telling him, just give me the word and we'll book the tickets back to Australia right away – he just smiles.

He won't eat anything savoury, that hasn't changed. It's all sugary sweet and he's happy with that—so am I. I once offered him a savoury muffin, and he looked at it like it was a personal betrayal. 'Where's the icing?' he asked, genuinely offended. We laughed for a good five minutes, and from then on, I never made that mistake again. It's sweets or nothing for Dad..

We generally have a lovely time together. Oftentimes, I bring one of my children, depending on their school or work schedules. It actually helps inject some humour and interest into lunches that would quite frankly be a bit dull at times. Dad is sweet, though, and a kindness has emerged that had been lost for a time, where he is delighted by the simplest of things. Always, our visits end with several hugs and kisses, and always, 'I love you.' I always want him to know he's not a burden, he matters, and I love him no matter what.

However, at age seventy-seven, my lovely father decided it was time to do something he hadn't done since 1974 – he shaved off his beard! Never in my wildest dreams did I think I would now be buying shaving cream, razors, etc. for Dad!

And so, a year into this new life of his, Dad is happy and content with his lot, so long as there is someone around to have a good debate with from time to time.

Some things just don't change!

6

Well, Fancy That!

"So Dad, guess what I did?"

"What's that love?"

"I wrote a book. I sent it to a Publisher, kind of on a whim while I was saving to self-publish."

"Really? Did you really write a book?"

"Yes, Dad, I really did."

"Well, fancy that!"

And so ensued a conversation about creativity, following our dreams and daring to take risks. Dad reminisced about the time he quit his job to go farming with nothing but an idea and tools. "You've got to leap sometimes, love," he said. "Even if there's no net." Something Dad certainly has done throughout his life. It was also quite startling that at times, he still had these moments of lucid clarity.

The irony for me is that I completely forgot about the submission until six weeks later. I wasn't expecting anything to come of it—maybe a polite rejection letter at best, or more likely, no reply at all when coming home from visiting Dad with my daughter. It was a cold, wintry day when I cleared the mailbox and saw that a large envelope had been sent to me from London. I thought it was odd because my daughter was back from London – who would be sending something to me?

I opened the envelope and was dumbfounded to see it was a Publishing Contract! I didn't have my glasses near me, so I checked with my girl, and amongst the screaming and crying, realised that yes indeed it was a Publishing Contract.

Dad was right all along – dreams do come true.

I took a couple of days to settle down and think it all through, read the contract and pray about it with my family. There was a strange mix of excitement and fear swirling inside me—what if I wasn't good enough, what if they'd made a mistake? Doubts whispered quietly in the background, but so did a sense of quiet calling, a nudge that maybe, just maybe, this was the right path opening up before me. I then knew I had one very important thing to do – I needed to take this contract down and show my father. Even in his state, I'm sure he would appreciate it.

I walked into the home and asked Dad if we could speak in his room. He took me in and we sat on the bed. I pulled out the green folder and let him look at its contents. I had a big, beaming smile on my face, and then Dad gasped. He couldn't find the words that he was feeling, so he put his hand on my arm, and in that moment, I felt the weight of every unsaid thing between us melt into that simple gesture. My throat tightened, and I had to blink back tears. It was as if time paused to let me fully feel the tenderness, the pride, and the unspoken love we had both longed for. He told me this was the best news and got misty-eyed. It was perfect. It was the perfect response. To know, really for the first time in my life ever, that my father was actually proud of something creative that I had done. That was the best gift for me.

He looked at me and kept saying, "Oh, oh, oh, I just want the best for you, darling. Oh, oh, oh, this is so wonderful!"

Yes, it was. The perfect moment—where all the other times had been so 'less than,' like the time he skimmed through my poetry with a critical nod —this time was simply put: perfect.

Well, fancy that!

7

The Man

To say music was in my father's blood is to say the Pope is Catholic – hello, very true indeed.

Dad was born with a song, but unfortunately, his song has never been heard. There was a story of an African tribe that always struck me. In it, a person would go away for some time and wait for a song that they would sing upon the birth of their child. When that child was born, they would hear the song, and then again at meaningful moments in their life. Upon their death, that song would be sung one last time, then never be heard of again. My father never sang the song that was imprinted upon his DNA. That to me is the ultimate tragedy of this man's life.

Here we are today with a man who not only won't play music anymore on a piano, but he demanded I sell all his musical gear for him, and so I did. I cried when I had to send everything off to the buyer; it was the end of an era.

Gone are the handwritten arrangements he had done over the years. I used to see them scattered across the old upright piano in our lounge—yellowing sheets full of neat staves, lyrical scribbles, and carefully notated harmonies. As a child, I thought it was magical, like watching music come to life right there in our living room. Now, it's hard to believe he denies ever writing them. Yet, my father had produced and arranged music, longer than I had been alive.

The other sadness that carries on is his incredible intellect. This was a man who, at his prime, was invited to join the Mensa Group – the minds of the most elite and intelligent in the world. He declined. The funny thing is, he didn't feel confident enough to join, just like he never felt confident in his performing and suffered debilitating stage fright during his whole career. And yet this is so much of who my father was. Brilliant and wonderful, handsome and kind, but for whatever reason, he only found his confidence in being married. I guess that is something of the norm for his generation?

Dad's life included becoming a private pilot, performing in a vocal group on television, working in the advertising world, opening a homebrew shop, operating a restaurant and becoming a farmer. Not to mention, having sung with some of the top names in the sixties and seventies, making records, and then having his own jazz band for many years.

As a private pilot, I grew up with a father who flew planes as a hobby and would often take us and various other friends and family up in a small plane, too. I thought that was normal for dads to do; turns out I was wrong!

Originally, Dad started his working life in the Advertising world, something my middle brother is a genius at. However, the call of music was too loud to stay bound to four walls for Dad. He ended up working during the day for the P&T (Post and Telegraph), climbing up and down poles all over Auckland

and the Hauraki Gulf. Music was for nighttime, and with it came a whole new world and some famously flamboyant new friends. Being the sixties, there was a major shift in the world, so away went the bow ties and Brylcreem, and in came the paisley shirts, platform shoes and long hair - and that was just Dad's wardrobe!

Dad would sing jingles and perform for the vocal group Happen Inn for four years on television. He also did a lot of writing, arranging and producing within the music industry. For me, I thought it was normal growing up in television and recording studios - apparently not.

Not too long after flirting with a small piece of land and continuing on in the music scene, Dad had a longing to become a farmer. And so, whilst working, he headed off on farmers' courses and in time, became one. Then, in his newfound enthusiasm, he had the brilliant idea (not!) of heading north to a decent-sized farm, family in tow. So, off we went and spent the following decade being a farming family in the back blocks of the Kaipara Harbour.

Next came the dalliance with home brewing, which eventually turned into an actual Home Brew shop in the local town. My parents turned the farm into a Jersey Stud for a while and eventually went into beef farming. This, in turn, freed them up to do some travelling, and so for the first time ever, they ventured over to the great land of Australia. This would be one of the many trips for them over the years.

Dad's dream took him to owning a food bar, aka Uncles, in our small town. Those in New Zealand remember the iconic takeaway bars that were open until 2am. Along with this came the music that Dad had turned his back on for thirteen years.

It was certainly odd for us children to have a piano in the house, and no one ever played it. The piano ended up in my room and was more like a hiding place and a storage space to keep all our vinyl records on, along with a mountain of clothes!

Somehow, the call of music resounded within Dad's soul, and he allowed himself to get involved in a Jazz band that had started in the local area. Little did any of us know that this would start a series of events that would lead our family into the greatest turmoil we had ever encountered.

You never forget when your parents ask you to sit down so they can talk with you. Dad did most of the talking, and the whole gist of it was that he had fallen out of love with my Mum, and so the two of them were going to separate. At twenty-four, my whole world literally fell apart. The battle lines were drawn, and the next couple of decades turned into war, then branching out into ice-cold silence. We kids and the grandchildren became the collateral damage.

Mum and Dad divorced - a day that will forever be etched into my memory, as I was the one to break the 'official news' to my mother.

Dad moved on with someone else and started his own Jazz band again, after all those years out of the music scene.

He bought into a restaurant with his sister and brother-in-law, a dream he'd always had, but unfortunately, the place bombed.

And so started a rift within the family that never would be fully repaired.

THE MAN

He was a big dreamer, and people alongside him believed in his dreams too.

Unfortunately, most of his dreams toppled, with varying degrees of fallout. And yet, in witnessing those collapses, I've come to understand that the courage to dream is its own kind of triumph. My father may not have achieved all he set out to do, but he never stopped reaching, and in that reaching, he showed us the beauty—and the cost—of living a life unafraid to imagine more.

8

The Old, The New

The Manager of the home sounded unusually tense on the other end of the line, her voice clipped and urgent. I could feel my stomach tighten as I gripped the phone, sensing something serious was coming—something that would turn our already delicate world upside down.

The database they used to monitor Dad's behaviour, attitude, physical health, and mental aptitude had spat out a reading that he was now in the top percentile of patients who needed Psycho-Geriatric care, and this facility was not registered to care for such patients.

"Your father is now staying here illegally and needs to be transferred to a Psycho-Geriatric facility as soon as possible. After all, the owner of this facility could be fined heavily for having your Dad stay on."

Can you believe this? So after an urgent phone call to my husband, I rang the Manager back and started gathering information, names, and numbers, determining just how much time I had to make this transition for Dad.

I'm so grateful for my husband. What a rock he has been. Just last week, when I sat sobbing on the kitchen floor after yet another stressful phone call, he simply knelt beside me and held my hand, saying, "We'll figure it out, together." What an adventure we've been on in this journey that we never asked for, and yet again, seemed to choose us. My brothers and I are truly indebted to him for his patience, kindness and mad sense of humour in some very trying times!

The day of the transition was truly awful. Dad was confused and agitated, asking repeatedly why we were moving him and where he was going. The staff at the old facility avoided eye contact, and packing his belongings felt rushed and clinical. Every step felt like a betrayal, even though we knew it was necessary. The air was thick with tension, and I carried a knot in my stomach the entire day, unsure if we were doing the right thing or simply the only thing we could. It also became apparent how neglectful the current home had been. I would normally have reported them to the authorities, but I had to pick and choose my battles wisely at this time. We discovered a lot of things that, for legal purposes, I won't divulge here.

Our saving grace was that a former staff member of the previous home was working at this new facility, which Dad was being admitted to. She literally walked out the front door as we were walking in, and Dad recognised her immediately. Her presence and care in those ensuing weeks are a kindness we can never repay her.

Upon entering the new ward, Dad was stunned to recognise a man he went to High School with and had even shared a hospital room with a few years prior. His eyes lit up in a way I hadn't seen in weeks, and he pointed, smiling widely and whispering, "That's Barry! We sat next to each other in class!" For a fleeting moment, the fog lifted—he stood taller, more sure of where he was, like he'd stumbled upon an old thread of himself. What were the chances of that??

After initially getting Dad into the facility, we were then advised it would be best to leave and let the team take over. Thankfully, the known carer came and spent the afternoon with Dad and helped him settle into his room.

There are moments of grace and peace we need to acknowledge and be thankful for.

There are moments of ourselves being scared, only wanting to hold our ailing father and tell him it's all going to be ok, he's not alone, and he never will be.

But for that moment, as our hearts break, our eyes leak—and somehow, even through the ache, we breathe. We remember that transition is not just loss, but possibility. He is safe, he is seen, and for now, that is enough to carry us into tomorrow. We sit with more paperwork to do, and we know that he will be fine for the time being.

9

Tom and Bruce

I was always struck by Tom. A dashing, handsome man, very well put together, usually sporting dress pants and a lovely red sweater. How he loved to dance, and when music came on in the room, Tom wanted to dance!

Dad's friend Tom was an absolute delight. The two of them were stuck together like glue at Dad's first home.

Tom did as Dad said, and therefore, Dad was happy! Their friendship was a mix of quiet understanding and shared routine—Dad loved to be in charge, and Tom didn't mind following suit. It became their unspoken rhythm: Dad giving directions, Tom nodding agreeably, both of them feeling purposeful in the process. There was something sweet about it, almost like watching two kids in a clubhouse, each playing their role with ease and affection.

But in reality, whilst Tom had Dementia, Tom was also very sick and wasn't going to be around for much longer.

Unfortunately, the last time Dad saw Tom, the latter was violently ill, slumped in his chair and barely able to acknowledge Dad's presence. It was a confronting and heartbreaking sight for

Dad, who stood silently for a long time, unsure of what to say or do. Later, he quietly told me, 'That's not my mate anymore,' his voice thick with sorrow. That final image lingered for days—Dad seemed quieter, more withdrawn, as if a part of his own joy had faded along with Tom's strength.

He missed his buddy, and to be honest, so did I.

RIP Tom. You brought much delight, friendship and smiley happy moments to Dad and the home, while you were there.

Bruce. He was a bit on the rough side, but with a kind and gentle heart. You could tell that Bruce had lived a colourful life, and that was evident in some of his storytelling! I remember one day he launched into a tale about hitchhiking across the country in the 70s to chase a woman he later admitted was "completely bonkers"—but he laughed so hard telling it, tears rolled down his cheeks. He had a rough edge, sure, but his warmth always came through in those twinkling eyes and his way of leaning in when he asked, 'How's your old man today?'

Dad and him would have the odd tiff, because Bruce wasn't compliant like Tom had been, but they were mates, and it was lovely to see.

My sadness is that Dad never got to say goodbye to Bruce, and was essentially whisked away to another home, care of the over-reaction of the Manager at the time (in another chapter).

At times, the lack of compassion and humanity is utterly horrendous. I had enquired as to whether I could bring Dad back to visit Bruce, and was told no. I remember being told, without any real explanation or empathy, that Dad wouldn't be allowed to return for a simple visit—no goodbye, no closure. It felt cold, like the system had no room for sentiment or dignity, just rigid protocol. Watching my father quietly process that absence broke something in me.

Fortunately, he would move into the home and be reunited with a former friend from High School - oh, the irony.

10

Going Back in Time

I guess I somehow felt triggered—maybe it was the sterile smell of disinfectant in the hallway or the sound of an old man coughing softly down the corridor—that instantly transported me back to when he first had to be put into a facility, and just the impact of that decision and the ensuing consequences.

The doctor had spoken to me after Dad's second but most 'official' diagnosis of Dementia. We would wait, and he would be assessed by a Gerontology Nurse who would come to his home and see what he needed assistance with. She would then report back to the authorities her recommendations, and for a while at least, he would still be in his own home but have the required help, and me.

Sounds good, but for one thing - Dad wasn't having a bar of it! He would go off shouting and demanding all sorts of things, then eventually calm down enough to listen to some sense of reason.

His wounds had healed, but his agitation levels were getting worse not by the week, but by the day. I would turn up to his place with morning tea or lunch, and he'd throw a fit. I'd gotten the food wrong, it was too hard, it was too soft, gosh, it went on and on. He used to go to the local bakery, and so I asked the owner, who was used to seeing him twice a day for months on end, what Dad ordered. I would then buy my choices according to that. But it was always wrong. I had to remind myself constantly that this was the Dementia at play and not my real Dad. But sometimes the verbal abuse just got too much.

After the Gerontology Nurse had visited a couple of times, it became apparent that although Dad had done an incredible job existing, he needed specialised care that wasn't going to come in the form of a couple of hours a week; he needed to be in a facility.

So we started looking, and to be honest, it was revolting. The stale smell of disinfectant, urine, and staff who barely looked up when we entered—it was soul-crushing. Some places felt more like warehouses than homes, and I left each one feeling nauseous and heartbroken. There was no way I was going to leave Dad in a place that felt so empty of warmth or dignity.. I shan't say here what I really felt at some of the facilities we saw, but needless to say, Dad wasn't going in there!

Dad needed to be monitored and thoroughly assessed, and the only way to do that was to have him committed to the Elderly Mental Health ward at North Shore Hospital. This is where the Enduring Power of Attorney over his health and well-being really came into play, and boy, was I grateful to have that piece of paper. People sit up and listen when you have that.

In order for anything to happen, we needed to have Dad 'sectioned'. A family meeting was held where two Mental Health Workers came to our home and laid out a plan. I didn't realise that they were wanting to do this today!

It ended up just being my husband and me who went around to talk with Dad, and then introduced him to the Workers. Since I had the Power of Attorney over his Health and Well-being, it was my decision ultimately as to whether Dad should go or not. After giving permission, it then became something I wasn't mentally or emotionally prepared for. Of course, Dad went off his tree and was demanding we all leave; he just wanted some lunch and a coffee. He was told that if he didn't go of his own free will, the local police would come and assist with this procedure. Well, that flicked him into another meltdown, to which he finally agreed. I asked him for his keys, told him I would come and see him tomorrow and that I loved him. He responded by yelling, "This is all your fault!"

And it was. I had given the okay for my Dad to be taken away 'by the men in white coats.' I nearly fainted on that driveway, groaning sobs in full, complete emotional overload.

They had taken my Daddy, and I couldn't protect him anymore.

Would he ever trust me again?

Argh, you never get over it really, seeing the look of fear and dread in your father's eyes. Hearing him yelling so loudly and then watching him drop his head in the back seat of the car. Alone and helpless.

He never entered that flat again.

To be honest, I don't remember getting back home that day. My husband somehow got me upstairs and into bed, and there I stayed on and off for five days. I did get up and go to the hospital, but I was on overdrive and robotic by then. I recall waking a few hours after going to bed that first afternoon and hearing a somewhat erratic conversation between my husband and my father on my mobile phone – I was very confused.

It seems that the hospital allowed the patients the occasional use of the phone, and when Dad got his hands on it, he used it with full gusto—dialling through like a man with a mission. It was both heartbreaking and slightly absurd to hear him, from the hospital, plotting his 'escape' and assigning us roles in the getaway. There was something surreal about it all, like a dark comedy unfolding in real time. That moment, though tinted with grief, reminded us of the sharp wit and stubborn will that still flickered within him. My husband decided, after trying to explain some things, to go along with Dad's plan, in theory! We've used this tactic many times since.

When I did go to the hospital, I was shocked to see Dad sitting quite happily chatting away to one of the other patients. This turned out to be his former High School friend, and now they were in an Elderly Mental Health ward together – serendipity? Either way, it was helpful to know that Dad had someone to chat with because at this stage, his long-term recall was far better than his short-term recall.

After my eldest brother flew to New Zealand, he became a great help with all of this. He had originally trained as a nurse, so he flicked straight back into that mode and spoke with the Medical Team in ways that I couldn't. Both my brothers protected and stood up against Dad when he was trying to go at me on one particular visit. Dad was let known this was a decision discussed and made by all three of his children, not just me, so that helped me a lot. It also made him calm the heck down.

11

Flat Memories

My first time going back into Dad's flat without him there was extremely emotional. For the first time, I could actually see just how Dad had set up his world in an ordered routine so that he could exist within his condition.

Firstly, I noticed his lists. They were everywhere: pinned on the fridge, taped beside the microwave, tucked near the radio and remote controls. Each one served a clear purpose: reminders for meals, how-to guides for appliances, and notes about his phone number. One listed his weekly grocery items, unchanged and familiar. Another detailed the steps to heat up his meals, despite identical instructions on the packaging. There were guides on using the computer, setting the radio alarm clock, and turning on the TV/DVD player. Scribbled in large writing, his new phone number was repeated on multiple scraps of paper. Near the phone, a list explained how to retrieve voice messages. Each note was a lifeline—an attempt to maintain order, independence, and clarity in a world increasingly clouded by confusion.

Next to his TV remotes and food tray was a table that had his viewing guide with all his favourite programmes circled, and his code-cracker books. Two of them, identical. They came out fortnightly, so he would do one, then buy it again the next week, do that and then go and buy a new issue the following week. My goodness, even in his addled mind, there still were elements of the genius he once had been.

I was afraid to touch anything. Somewhere deep in my mind, I had thought that perhaps they would release him, and so I decided not to do anything other than check that his food hadn't gone off. It wasn't until after speaking to one of the doctors at the hospital that I realised my Daddy wasn't ever coming home.

Queue more tears.

When I did finally have the gumption to start attacking his flat, it was on my own. In fact, the only help I was given was from Dad's former wife and the offer of help from his former stepdaughter. No one else offered, no one else came. It was all on me. Everything changed at that moment; former grudges, unforgiveness, pain, family 'loyalty' – it all ended that day.

When you sit in a cold, dark flat surrounded by papers, possessions, and the remnants of seventy-plus years of a life, the truth hits you hard. Truth comes and shows you things you may not want to see and hear, but eventually, truth and knowing the truth will ultimately set you free.

Looking through the many boxes of photos, memories came rushing back into my mind. I remember many different times when I could never live up to the impossibly high expectations he had of me. The constant attacks on my choices in life. The inane critique of any effort I would make at trying to be creative.

He was always criticising my outward appearance, always warning me to be 'good' and never allowing me to be anything other than his version of me. As I looked back, many different emotions would flood through me.

Seeing all the cards, pictures, letters and documents that were passed down through the generations. The beautifully framed photographs of my Nana's family when she was a gorgeous young girl with long blonde ringlets in her hair. My great-grandfather looked all dark and handsome, his Irish eyes staring out at us above a large bushy moustache. Her equally handsome older brothers looking back at me, and I almost felt guilty looking through all this stuff!

But then, how was I supposed to react, reading Dad's former will, knowing that he thought so very little of me, that he left me virtually nothing, and the best of what he had was going to my brothers? Here I was, the only child sorting out his affairs, and he thought that of me? Wow, what an ass he had been when he made that former will. It was pain upon pain, the realisation that my worst fears were real and I had been right all along. His beloved middle son, the apple of his eye, the one I was constantly compared to and could never live up to – where was he now? And the wild one, the eldest son whom Dad could never quite understand, where was he? That's right, they weren't here. I was.

And that had to mean something.

To Dad, it came to mean everything.

12

Back to the Present

After a while, normality set back into Dad and his new home, and we changed the day that I would go and visit him. Now I had three keypad-coded doors to walk through to get to my father. Each one felt like a barrier, not just of security, but of time and reality. The metallic beeps and clicks echoed as I moved through the quiet, carpeted hallways—clean, thoughtfully decorated, and filled with the gentle hum of friendly conversation. Though the environment was warm and the staff truly wonderful, the coded doors still felt symbolic, marking a transition into a new chapter of Dad's life—one that carried both care and constraint. Every door I opened felt like another step deeper into a version of him I was still learning to accept.

For the longest time, my Aunty would pick up Dad on a Saturday morning, take him out with her husband for morning tea, and then go back to their place so that Dad could watch some pre-recorded TV programmes. Unfortunately, due to some unforeseen circumstances, this now no longer happens.

I feel a huge sense of responsibility that Dad is taken out at least once a week. I've noticed that these outings seem to lift his spirits in ways that nothing else does. He becomes more animated—his eyes brighter, his smile quicker to form. Even a short drive or a simple café lunch seems to reawaken something familiar in him, like a spark of the man we've known and loved all our lives. It reminds me that these small moments aren't small at all; they're essential. I know it seems like I've taken on too much at times, and I could be misconstrued as going overboard, but he's our father. Any time that we have left with him should be celebrated and seen as a blessing rather than anything else. Dad and us children have had a checkered past for sure, but as far as I am concerned, that all went by the wayside upon his committal. It's that simple.

You should have seen Dad's face when I showed him my newly published book—his eyes went wide with wonder, then filled with tears. He held it in both hands like it was something sacred, his fingers tracing the cover as he whispered, "You did it, love." For a moment, he seemed completely present, as if nothing else in the world existed. It was as though all the years between us dissolved into that single look of pride and awe. I didn't think he'd want a copy as he can't concentrate enough to read now, so I took it home with me. My mistake. When I saw him the next week (I'd left the book in my handbag), he asked if he could possibly have one and if I could write in it, please? I truly feel like that's been one of the greatest honours of my life, knowing that it meant so much to Dad. Wonders will never cease!

We go to the same place to eat, and then he likes to go for a drive. My daughter made a playlist with all the kinds of music her Poppa likes, and so we put that on. Dad doesn't miss a beat.

He sings away and claps his hands, slaps his legs to the beat, and insists I sing too – luckily, I can sing.

At first, I found it hard to do all of this. I had so much anger, and the father that I would have usually had it out with, no longer exists. The turning point came one sunny afternoon as we sat in the car after lunch, he humming along to the music, smiling out the window. I looked over and saw not the man who had hurt me, but someone fragile and fading, still full of life in fleeting moments. Something inside me shifted. I had to make peace with the past and move into the present. God knows we're not promised tomorrow, so I really do try and make every visit count.

I grieve. Openly and honestly. But through the grieving, I've also found unexpected peace. This journey has taught me to treasure presence over perfection, grace over grudges. Somehow, in the quiet in-between moments, I've gained a deeper understanding of love—the kind that stays, even as memories fade. I grieve all the dreams that won't come true and the fact that the father I need is long gone. I wonder if he ever truly was there – I don't know. I just know that I've been given this time and that everything has been said that needs to be said. Every transgression, on both sides, has been forgiven.

Much love exudes from Dad, even though he steadily loses more and more vocabulary. He says lovely things and gets such a thrill when we turn up every week. It's like he is constantly surprised, and that is really sweet. And perhaps that's what this season is teaching me—not to wish for the past or fear the future, but to meet each moment with open hands. Every visit is a gift. And for now, that's enough.

13

Where Everybody Knows Your Name

The old television series 'Cheers' theme song has been on my mind a bit lately. In the lyrics, there is the line, "where everybody knows your name". That rings so true and loudly for me.

Being known and being seen are such an integral part of the human experience. People want to be known, they want to be acknowledged, they want to be greeted, and they want to feel validated. A lot of this is acknowledged when we show up, greet a person, and call them by their name. It makes a difference. It means something.

Until they forget your name.

Yesterday was such a day for me. The man who gave me my name could no longer remember it. The man who sang over me when I was born could no longer sing it. The man who calls me 'his world' forgot who I was. The man who lights up like a moonbeam when he sees me doesn't know if I am his wife, mother, or daughter.

Of course, the girls (my adult daughters) were with me, so that helped tremendously. Especially when your eldest is in the back of the car, squealing with delight at seeing the newborn lambs, and then mimics their 'baaaaa' full force, causing her Poppa to laugh - belly laugh! It helps me to know that I am not alone in this. My children and my husband are feeling it too. Although he remembers my 'tall' son and what his name is. And that stings strangely—how selective memory chooses one face and not another. It's both comforting and heartbreaking, watching him hold onto fragments while others, like my name, slip away. It reminds me that love doesn't always follow logic, and memory is a fickle, tender thing. He remembers my husband for his belly and his work ute. Dad is a card indeed!

I haven't actually released a blog on Dementia and the horrible effects of it since last year. I was determined that I wasn't going to write any more about it, but it turns out this is my catharsis, and I need to get this out of me before grief consumes the good in my world.

Make no mistake, I am grieving. I have been for over three years now. But the grief has changed shape. It started as disbelief, turned to guilt, then frustration, and finally—something quieter. Not easier, just softer. I've learned that grieving someone who's still alive requires a different kind of endurance, one that asks you to let go without turning away. I have been utterly consumed with guilt for being the child who had to lock up her Dad. I am through that now, but there were days when it was all-consuming. "Why did it have to be me? Why aren't the boys (my brothers) more involved? Why don't they check up on me and see how I am doing with all of this? Why do I have to be the one who does everything for Dad? Why, why, why?"

It's a vicious circle, one that embitters the soul and causes great anxiety, depression, and the propensity to make one harsh and demeaning. I can't afford any of that anymore. People will only do what they want to do and no more.

I am deeply saddened that I often find Dad in his room in complete disarray now. I sometimes have to remind him to finish getting changed. I am saddened that his pride and arrogance still lurk in the deepest recesses of his brain, and he is unable to ask for help with his self-care. It is this very issue that has caused the greatest stress and challenges in his life. The very reason that he's in the ward called Psycho-Geriatric. With the most aggressive and physically violent Dementia patients. And yet Dad is usually so kind and gentle. Remnants of a bygone era where Dad's winning personality and smile caused him to get away with blue murder!!

So, as much as I grieve and cry over the fact that Dad doesn't remember my name, I am deeply grateful that I still can put a smile on his face, and that he loves me.

Maybe that's what the song was really about—not just knowing names, but being known in the moments that matter most. In the end, all we have is love – and that's enough.

14

The Bin

His clothes had been disappearing, and I started noticing Dad wearing items that clearly weren't his own.

At first, I wasn't sure what to make of it—there was a moment of confusion, even a flicker of absurd humour. But when I looked in his wardrobe and saw the stack of unfamiliar clothes and blankets, a quiet sadness settled in. It was like finding a secret he hadn't meant to keep, a signpost pointing to how much further he had drifted into his own world. It turned out that when his clothes became soiled in any way, he would tie them up in a bundle and throw them in the bathroom bin. His other method? Stuffing them into his mattress! I didn't even know he could unzip the protective mattress cover—but clearly, he's still a smart cookie in some areas.

That's when I realised: Dad had developed a new problem. It caught me off guard—I couldn't help but laugh at the sheer absurdity of it, even while a lump formed in my throat. It was one of those moments where humour and heartbreak collided, and I found myself both chuckling and grieving at the same time. He'd become a kleptomaniac. It sounds funny, and in some moments, it is, but it was serious enough that the home had to start locking cupboards, bedrooms, and wardrobes. Dad was on the prowl!

He had amassed a huge stack of beautifully folded bath towels, facecloths, and hand towels—nineteen full sets, all neatly arranged. The staff had been scratching their heads, wondering why the ward was running low on towels. One nurse even joked with me, "We thought we had a towel thief, but we didn't expect it to be your dad with a full linen department in his wardrobe!" We laughed, but underneath it was this odd mixture of pride and heartbreak. Dad's stash had been folded so neatly, as if part of him still craved purpose and control. Well, now we knew. Of course, when they removed the stash, Dad accused them of stealing. This pattern went on for months.

At Dad's stage of Dementia, he's still lucid enough to make these choices, and convincing enough to make staying ahead of him quite difficult.

I've had to replace so many items—clothes, shoes, belts, toiletries. The home now hides several sets of his clothing, so there's always something clean and fresh for him after his showers. Right now, he tries to wear three jumpers and seven polo shirts, all at once. At first, we tried reasoning with him or gently removing a few layers, but he'd get defensive or agitated. These days, the staff and I mostly let it go unless it poses a health risk. It seems to bring him comfort, and in a world that no longer makes sense to him, who are we to take that away?

The latest change? After years of wearing the exact same style of sneaker, Dad now only wants to wear his slippers. That's fine—we let him go out in whatever makes him feel comfortable. The other issue is a bit trickier: sometimes he removes his pull-ups and refuses to wear them. We now keep a towel in the car. Just in case. Good grief. And an extra set of clothes. Thankfully, we've not had to use them, yet!

Despite all of this, Dad still loves to sit and sing his heart out. He's so sweet and kind. I don't often see his aggressive side, though I do get phone calls when he lashes out at other residents or staff. To manage this, his sedative medication has been increased significantly.

I often wonder how things might be different if we had Dementia Villages here in New Zealand. The idea of a place that feels more like a neighbourhood than a facility: a place where Dad could safely roam, garden, or pop into a familiar-looking café, deeply appeals to me. I think he would thrive in an environment designed to gently mirror normal life, where dignity and routine are woven into every detail. It feels like such a hopeful and compassionate model of care.

I'm often struck by the contrast in residents: some run around causing mayhem, while others are confined to chairs or beds. The staffing is limited, but the staff are genuinely incredible. Dad may give them 'what for' at shower time, but he truly does love them. He considers them friends.

My father's body and heart seem built for longevity, but his mind has steadily declined.

Though the grieving has softened, I still miss him a lot.

But God be praised, he's still here. Still wonderfully responsive.

If only he would stop throwing his clothes away!

15

Three Minutes Fifty-One

One week before New Zealand entered total Lockdown, the Rest Homes and Aged Care facilities made an early decision: they would close their doors to visitors to protect their vulnerable residents. At the time, we were led to believe that the Coronavirus, COVID-19 or SARS-CoV-2, was most lethal towards the elderly and infirm. Unfortunately for our country, this proved to be true. Most of our small cases of deaths were indeed in the Rest Homes.

Dealing with not seeing Dad was something that I was consciously aware of when our Prime Minister started to make daily addresses to the public regarding the Lockdown. Then the day hit when I realised there would be no visiting him at all, and I didn't get the chance to warn him. However, all was not lost, as I was able to speak to him on the phone, and the home was able to arrange a couple of Skype calls.

Dad was actually quite funny on those Skype calls; he'd squint at the screen, wave enthusiastically, and ask, "How did you all get inside that little box?" At one point, he tried to reach forward to touch the screen and accidentally ended the call, which had us all laughing. His confusion was endearing, and his delight at seeing our faces, no matter how surreal it seemed to him, was unmistakable. The whole conversation lasted three minutes and fifty-one seconds.

Yes folks, that three minutes and fifty-one seconds really put all my fears to rest. (Insert dry sarcasm here.) In reality, it was both comforting and painfully inadequate, a bittersweet moment that highlighted just how much we were all grasping for reassurance.

When I was able to visit Dad eventually after ten weeks, I had to go through a whole routine of sanitisation, form filling, and mask-wearing. Dad didn't even realise it was me until I quickly lifted the mask up so he could see my entire face!

He understood that I wasn't able to take him out, and instead of focusing on his own disappointment, he immediately turned his attention to me. Ever the protective father, even in his diminished state, he grew agitated that other residents were approaching me. He kept trying to shoo them away, telling one, "Go away, get away from us!" It was touching and funny—this glimpse of his old self, still trying to look after me in the only way he could.

I have to say, in this instance, there were so many unprecedented things happening in our world, but I learned not to worry about Dad. The staff again were utterly brilliant and would keep us informed with emails, texts and the occasional photographs of Dad. He was being entertained and kept busy, which relieved a whole lot of pressure off of me.

In hindsight, that season taught me something lasting: even when the world feels uncertain, love finds a way to reach through. Whether through a pixelated smile, a protective outburst, or a thoughtfully shared photo, connection still endures. And for that, I exhale deeply and smile.

16

Hands

I was just sitting in the back of the car while my husband drove. Dad sat in the front, singing his heart out to Frank Sinatra. I was remembering. Times spent with Dad, in the home and the trips that we frequently take him on.

One such time, we went to Waiwera, a lovely seaside village north of Auckland, and found ourselves in an area that was not too familiar to me. It was along a single road, on the beachfront, but in an area that was quite private. We parked the car, and I helped Dad out. It was a lovely sunny day, so we ventured onto the beach. However, Dad seemed a bit unstable, so I held his hand to steady him.

It was odd. I hadn't held Dad's hand like that since I was sixteen years old, back when we used to walk down the main road of the town we once lived in. Somewhere along the line, the comfort of that connection faded into adulthood, replaced by a kind of emotional distance I hadn't realised was there, until suddenly, in that moment, it wasn't. One remembers these things. The moments when subtle little changes became the norm, and holding hands with your father was no longer the 'done' thing.

But on this particular day, he needed me. And I was there, steadying him, guiding him, offering back the kind of gentle assurance he once gave me as a child. It was a quiet shift, tender and humbling, stepping into the role of caretaker. A part of me resisted it, aching for the man who never used to need help. But another part, deeper and softer, felt honoured to be trusted with his hand. I guess the little girl in me needed him at that moment, too. It didn't last long, but it was just us - just a special moment in our collective history that will always remain with me.

Walking through the home, alongside hubby, I held Dad's hand again today. The linoleum floors gleamed under the overhead lights, and the faint scent of chemical cleaning spray lingered in the air. We passed the common room where a quiet game of cards was in progress, and the walls were dotted with cheerful artwork painted by residents. It was familiar and warm, yet still slightly disorienting, especially today. He was a little nervous, as we had to walk a different way than usual, but he gripped my hand as I led him through the maze of hallways.

He can't think of much to say at the moment, but he does remark time and again, how much he enjoys being with hubby and me. It's lovely. His shock of hair standing on end, his teeth seemed to have moved, and he's developed a lisp now. His hands, like my Nana's, are bony and slender—familiar in a way that stirred something deep inside me. I remembered sitting beside her as a child, tracing the veins along the back of her hand with my finger, the same way I now noticed Dad's. There was comfort in that symmetry, like touching history twice.

His appetite seems to have returned, which is a big relief.

| 60 | - HANDS

    My Dad.
Bony hands and all.
How I love him.

17

The Father

I knew, walking into the theatre, that I was setting myself up for an emotional rollercoaster. I expected the tears, the rawness, and the weight of what was to come. And I wasn't wrong. But it turns out, they weren't mine. Well, not till the last five minutes, and then I felt myself crack.

To my left was a young couple who found the content too much and left partway through the movie, utterly sobbing. With all of the best intentions, I wanted to go to that young lady and tell her it was okay, that she wasn't alone. I wanted to give her a hug and tell her I completely understand, but essentially, I don't.

You see, for each of us who are the child of a Dementia sufferer, there are coping mechanisms we have formed. There are emotions we won't show. There are areas where our experiential expertise doesn't cover. Therefore, whilst we should have empathy and compassion for all concerned, we shouldn't go butting our imposter noses into others' suffering. We need to be *invited into the suffering* and then offer ourselves to the one hurting. That invitation might come in the form of a shared story, a quiet moment of eye contact, or a simple request for company—any signal that the person is ready to be met where they are.

The movie, 'The Father', is a brilliant portrayal of a Dementia sufferer, through his own eyes. I clicked onto that notion within a couple of scenes at the beginning of the movie. As the storyline unfolded, evidence of my own Dad came raring to the forefront, and I was left feeling somewhat vindicated.

The nonstop comparisons. The nitpicking. The angry outbursts of swearing and cursing. The silent treatment. The endless demands. The accusations of being up to no good. These are all things that my Dad heaped on me, time and time again. Fortunately, I have a wonderful husband, great brothers and a mother with the patience of a Saint - although, since long divorced from my Dad, still a loving friend and a great listening ear for me.

If any of you are either curious or have a loved one battling Dementia or Alzheimer's, then I thoroughly encourage you to see this movie. It helps tremendously. It gives such a compelling insight into the mind of a former intellect, who is now at the mercy of this dreaded affliction. Anthony Hopkins gives a stellar performance, bringing all the pain, emotion and frustration right towards you. You can't duck and avert it; you have to experience it right to the end, and then the ending leaves you speechless.

I was somewhat mortified at the conclusion of the movie, when I had to go to the bathroom. Many of us were heading there to reapply our cried-off makeup. Upon entering, I heard some women laughing at said movie, and how they would love to end up with Dementia when they were older. Well, suffice it to say, I was deeply upset. Their flippant remarks felt like a slap in the face after such a raw and moving experience. It was hard not to let the anger take over, but I also knew it came from a place of ignorance, more than anything else. After being in an already emotional state, the thought of bumping into them and having to make small talk, when in reality I wanted to punch them for their insensitive and erroneous remarks, was enough to make me get out of there fast! Their mockery, I pray, will not become their self-fulfilling prophecy.

A few days after seeing that movie, I walked into Dad's Dementia unit, and there he was, sitting, having a cup of tea and biscuits. His hair sticking up like a scarecrow, runny nose and scruffy jumper aside, the smile that greets you is immense. He's like a kid in a candy store, and he knows he's about to have a lot of candy! Always the question, "Are we going out now for something to eat, then a drive up north?" Always, a kiss and hug and the words, "You're the best thing in the world." Of course, I am; I'm the Sugar Fairy and Taxi operator!

Coming back from our afternoon excursion, I was shocked to see a formerly vibrant and active resident, now needing a carer on both sides, to assist her walking. Colleen was a gummy bear who refused to wear her teeth, could swear like a trooper, and propositioned my husband upon meeting him the first time! Her antics made us laugh more than once, but behind the humour was a woman grappling with her own decline. It reminded me how much personality still flickers within, even as memory fades. She loved dancing and could flirt up a storm; if only in her own mind. It was nothing for her to stroke my arm and do a little jig with me, then start weeping. On the flipside, she could spot me across the room and start marching towards me, yelling expletives, and promising to "get me!"

My heart is saddened, for I know the day will come when my Dad will need that kind of help, too.

In the meantime, when he sits in the café with us, his latest fixation is on the 'Fire Exit' sign, alongside the 'Toilets' sign.

His most recent revelation? "Toilets are where you go poos and wees!!"

18

As Time Goes By...

Where are you?
Did life simply move on, or did the silence grow too loud??
Why have you stopped visiting Dad?
How long since you've been in touch with him?
Have you tried calling or Skyping?
It never ceases to amaze me—the tender justifications people create to ease their own discomfort when avoiding someone with Dementia. I try to understand it, but it still hurts.
The list is endless, and I too, have used some of those excuses, but in reality, they don't work.
Where are the friends Dad used to have? You know, the ones he would meet up with regularly, at a cafe or in their home.
Where are the ones who, upon his committal, promised me they'd always stay in touch?
Who said they'd only be a phone call away??
Why are my brother and I the only ones who bother to see Dad now?

It's bloody hard, it really is. Hard when you walk into his room and he doesn't know your name. Hard when you say goodbye and wonder if it's the last time. Hard when you sit beside him and talk to the silence that used to be your father.

But, as time goes by, so does the necessity to keep one's word.

Ah, this world is fickle, full of people who once brought casseroles and comfort, now too busy to reply to a message or make a call.

Life is fleeting.

But in some cases, it seems to go on and on.

But, I do wonder, where are you?

19

The Manager

My goodness, this year has certainly had some curveballs in store for us!

We experienced a couple of small lockdowns near the beginning, and then we experienced a very long, arduous one on my mother's 80th birthday. Not ideal. Of course, we were kept in the loop with Dad's Care Home, all the way through, but there were some big changes to navigate.

Firstly, I was told I had to be double vaccinated to see my father, which caused me some great anxiety. In the end, we all chose to be vaccinated, along with Dad, but I didn't appreciate being put into a corner. This should have been my choice, not a blanket threat. I understand they were doing their best in difficult circumstances, trying to protect the most vulnerable, but it was still a confronting and painful decision to be forced into. However, what's done is done, and that particular manager has moved on.

We endured 107 days in lockdown, here in the Auckland area. Fortunately, we were able to speak to Dad on the phone and Skype with him. He responded very well this time and didn't get up and walk away from the computer, as he had done in times past.

Dad is now 82, so his desire to be gone before 80 didn't come true. For that, we are truly thankful.

By and large, Dad's thoughts and vocabulary have been reduced to what he wants to eat, going in the car and going back to his 'work'. It seems he can't think of his Care Home as a 'home', but he sees it as his 'work'. The irony is, at times, he is called 'The Manager'! He likes to dictate where people can and can't sit within the large dining room and lounge, and if he doesn't want the windows or curtains open in there, he will follow the staff around as they open them and shut them. My father, he makes me laugh so much! He's also taken to drinking other people's hot drinks when they're not looking, and then, at times, throws the cups out the window! Dad loves hiding as many cups, plates and bibs in cupboards, where he thinks no one will find them. He honestly never stops surprising me.

He no longer seems to resist showers and toileting now, but he does get up occasionally in the middle of the night and insist it's breakfast time - oh Dad!

He still seems to do what I call, 'go shopping' within his ward, and is wearing a lovely hat that wasn't bought for him. Cheese cutter in style, it's similar to one that he wears, which used to belong to his father, my delightful poppa. He still has issues wearing his belt, because he's always losing it, along with his wallet, his combs, brushes and the like. Still, on the odd times I have been into his room this past year, I have noticed a lot of mail he's been keeping that he's never opened. It made me wonder—was he confused, overwhelmed, or simply avoiding the reality those envelopes might contain? Perhaps it was a quiet protest against a world that kept shifting around him, or maybe he just didn't want reminders of what he could no longer fully grasp. I tried to help him with that, but he always resisted. Also, I happened to notice that he had acquired several CDs and DVDs that I know aren't his. Yes, my father likes 'shopping'!

He no longer recognises his grandchildren, but in an interesting irony, he recognises photos of them as little children, and photos of himself in previous decades. His memories of a bygone era, whilst needing a jolt at times, still seem to be there.

We still spend a lot of time singing Frank Sinatra, Dean Martin and Michael Bublé in the car. Those songs have become a bridge between us—a shared rhythm that cuts through the fog of his memory. Each verse brings back glimpses of the man he was and still is in fleeting moments, and for me, they are treasured echoes of our past.

My father still has the voice of an angel, and I am so fortunate that I get to hear him sing.

20

Twenty Twenty-Three!

My, how the world has transformed since my initial writings about Dad and our journey through dementia. Rereading those early entries, it feels like an eternity since the day we made the difficult decision to have Dad committed and placed into a care home. At the time, it felt like heartbreak cloaked in necessity—a mix of guilt, grief, and relief. Now, looking back, I realise it was an act of love in one of its hardest forms. The road since then has been tumultuous, and there's still more to come.

Presently, Dad sports an unshaven look, his hair resembling Albert Einstein's wild mane. It's both amusing and heartbreaking—amusing because it suits his once-playful defiance, and heartbreaking because it highlights just how far we've drifted from the man who once took such pride in his appearance. He prefers the lounge near the television for his nightly sleep, maintaining his authority over the remote control. No channel changes are permitted without his explicit permission - a quirk that doesn't surprise me.

He has a companion who sits beside him, engaging in conversations that I can only imagine, as Dad's thoughts are now scattered. His feet bear the toll of diabetes and lack of movement, making their care a significant undertaking. Attending to them involves regular checks for sores, careful trimming of toenails, and ensuring circulation remains stable—all tasks that feel more intimate and sobering than I ever anticipated. Each time I see them, I'm reminded of how vulnerable he has become, and how much diligence and compassion are required in the smallest acts of care. Dad's two front teeth are now absent, and he adamantly refuses any attempt to clean or approach them. It's a stark contrast to the man he once was.

Dad still engages in his peculiar 'shopping' ritual, donning clothes and a fedora hat that doesn't belong to him. I find myself spending a considerable amount replacing his wardrobe as he continues to gain weight, a silver lining in this challenging situation.

Taking him out has become a rarity; recognition of us seems to have slipped away, and he prefers staying in his chair. It's a quiet, painful shift—one that has forced me to recalibrate what connection looks like. I've learned to meet him where he is, to find comfort in holding his hand or simply sitting beside him in silence. The absence of recognition doesn't erase our bond; it just reshapes it. I respect his choices, avoiding any imposition. However, I continue to bring him biscuits and chocolate, encouraging him to sing.

Moments of joy emerge when I share photos of him with our family, bringing a fleeting smile to his face.

Several times, there have been the type of phone calls, where all I can do is apologise for Dad's behaviour. It seems that he has grown a penchant for throwing things in people's faces, like cups, glasses and plates. Thank God, there haven't been any serious injuries, but it is very disheartening to hear. Dad also pushes people over if they get too close to him - literally. He doesn't like anyone getting in his personal space without asking, and he will certainly let you know!

Fortunately, the staff have been wonderful at navigating these incidents, and assure me this is all part of the disease.

21

My Way

This year, 2024, although only in the month of March, has already brought a cascade of health challenges for our beloved father, including a bout of cellulitis, a heart attack, and what appeared to be a mild stroke.

There have been a few times that Dad ended up in the hospital, and we were shocked at how quickly he declined into a new level of helplessness.

It seems our father had a case of cellulitis in one of his legs, which brought on a heart attack. Back at the home, there were good and bad days. It seemed to my brother and me that he had endured a mild stroke, as his left side seemed weak and droopy. Dad also could no longer walk, and was put in a recliner and kept out in the lounge during the day. That then changed, and he was in his room quite a bit now, resting. The phone calls from the home were becoming more frequent, and there were more and more decisions having to be made.

I also decided, since Dad was spending a lot of time asleep in his room, to put up photos of the family, his sisters, parents and all the grandchildren, all over the walls. In some way, I wanted him to know we were all there, and he wasn't alone.

Then we had 'the' phone call. I lost it completely. After all these years, and with everything that I've walked through with my Dad, I wasn't ready for him to go. Purely selfish, but I needed him just a little while longer. There were still things I longed to say, memories to revisit, and simple, quiet moments I wasn't yet ready to release. I needed his presence, his familiar face, his voice, even if he didn't fully recognise mine.

The children came and said goodbye, and I arranged for some other family members to come the following day.

He seemed to have a resurrection! And he was yelling at them to 'get out!' Oh dear...

I was with him after that phone call, which obviously was premature, and I was helping feed him. The carer for one of the other residents started chatting with me, and I commented that we'd been on this journey for nearly eight years. Suddenly, Dad said, "Have I really been here for eight years?"

"Yes, Dad, you have."

"But I can't remember any of it!"

"It's okay Dad, we all have days when we can't remember things."

The look of sadness was too much for me, so as I turned to wipe some escaping tears, I opened a box of chocolates and offered him one. His eyes lit up, a gentle smile curved on his lips, and he reached out with surprising eagerness. It was a small flicker of joy that pierced the heaviness of the moment, and I clung to it.

A few weeks later, I got another one of 'those' phone calls.

My husband and I arranged to meet with my brother at the home.

They had left him in his bed this time, and he was very weak, his breathing very shallow.

This time, we knew. We spent the day with him, stroking his hair, holding his hands, whispering quiet prayers, and quietly chatting with others who popped in.

He was getting ready to fly.

We looked into those beautiful blue eyes and bid him farewell, amongst our tears and groans. Whilst looking straight at us, a single tear fell from his eye. I kissed his forehead, we all did, and told him he had many waiting for his homecoming, so it was time to leave. With a quiet breath, he was gone.

Dad slipped into eternity.

It was beautiful and peaceful.

True to his life's song 'My Way' by Frank Sinatra, Barry William Clewett did indeed do things his way. Right up to the end, he charted his own course.

Godspeed Dad. Until we meet again...

22

The Final Chapter

In the weeks following Dad's passing, I surprised myself with how well I was holding up. The memorial, though heartfelt, didn't quite unfold the way I'd hoped—but it was done with love, and it honoured him in all the ways that mattered.

Seven weeks later, I found myself overseas on a Solidarity Mission to Israel—a journey I never imagined would come so soon after saying goodbye. That trip deserves a story of its own, filled with moments of awe, challenge, and unexpected clarity. But at the time, I was still moving forward, still in motion, and still not fully registering the weight of what had passed.

It wasn't until November 2024, months later, that the real grief arrived. Not like a thunderclap, but a slow, creeping tide. After nine years of walking through the Dementia journey, of bracing myself for every twist and loss, the silence that followed his passing was deafening. I thought I was okay. I told myself I was okay. But I wasn't.

I stopped writing. I stopped creating. I stopped doing anything that asked for a part of my heart. I poured myself into my family and into healing. I learned to breathe again—slowly, deliberately. I gave myself permission to just be. To cry. And I did—every single day for months.

And then, one day, I didn't.

That was the day I turned a corner. Not a finish line, but a bend in the road. A soft place where grief and acceptance could sit side by side.

Dad still comes to me in dreams. Sometimes he's himself again. Other times, he still needs help. It's strange and tender and unresolved. Perhaps I'll always carry some part of this journey with me. Perhaps that's the cost of love.

Dementia is a thief. A robber of clarity, of independence, of shared memories. It twists the narrative and muddles the edges of everything familiar. But what it can't take are these moments; these memories I've written down, the photos, the videos, the sound of his voice tucked away in recordings. He's not lost to us. Not truly.

I do miss the old boy. Fiercely. But I know, deep in the marrow of my bones, that he is in heaven, surrounded by the family that went before him. I picture him on the balconies of glory, watching over us, cheering us on.

That thought gives me peace. And breath. And strength for all the chapters still to come, in this crazy, mixed up and yet amazingly beautiful thing we call life.

23

Help!

When this journey began, the signs of Dementia weren't immediately apparent to me, aside from the more obvious indicators like memory loss. It became clear that everyone's experience with Dementia is unique, but there are key observations to consider when navigating this challenging path with loved ones.

Early Signs to Watch Out For:
A proliferation of lists and rigid adherence to routines.
Forgetting simple names and places that should be easy to recall.
Unexplained outbursts of anger.
A seeming emotional detachment, contrary to their past behaviour.
Laughing at serious matters.
Muddling up stories and memories.
Saying NO to everything.
Needing help with personal care and hygiene.
Avoiding people in their homes despite past sociability.

Becoming gruff, rude, arrogant, and aggravated compared to their usual calm demeanour.

Eating issues, possibly leading to malnourishment and dehydration.

Clenched fists.

Comparing loved ones to each other becomes a recurrent behaviour.

While there are many potential symptoms, these stood out vividly in my experience. Recognising them early made all the difference—it allowed me to seek support sooner and better prepare for the journey ahead.

Seeking Support:

If you find yourself grappling with these signs, don't hesitate to seek support. Local nurses and doctors can offer valuable insights, and reaching out to them is a good starting point. Short, focused conversations with professionals can provide guidance, and they may share contacts for further discussions.

Support Groups and Resources:

Explore support groups for caregivers of dementia patients. These communities offer a wealth of shared experiences and practical advice. Additionally, online resources can be valuable, providing information and connecting you with a broader community.

Reaching Out to Others:

Connect with individuals like ministers, pastors, vicars, elders, counsellors, or trusted friends. They can offer emotional support and may have access to resources not readily available through hospitals.

Navigating Care Facilities:
When your loved one enters a care facility, engage with the staff. Identify those who build a strong bond with your loved one and can navigate the evolving circumstances. Asking for help is not a sign of weakness but a crucial step in managing this journey.

Family Involvement:
Involve your family, siblings, and trusted friends, but be aware that they may be as unfamiliar with the situation as you are. Everyone's journey is unique, and shared support can be beneficial.

Additional Resources in New Zealand:
For those in New Zealand, the Alzheimer's Association offers valuable information, including the option to join the 'Dementia Friend' program: www.alzheimers.org.nz/explore/dementia-friendly-nz/become-a-dementia-friend/

Faith and Coping:
As a Bible-believing Christian, my faith was a cornerstone during the dark days. Prayer became a daily lifeline, and Scripture offered comfort when words failed me—verses like Psalm 34:18 reminded me that the Lord is close to the brokenhearted. Faith can be a sustaining force, providing strength through challenging

times. It's important to acknowledge that, ultimately, for Dementia sufferers, death becomes a form of freedom.

While we may be fortunate to have our loved ones with us for an extended period, still leading a relatively good life, these moments are treasures to be cherished.

In writing these blogs, I hope these insights provide both practical guidance and a sense of shared understanding for those navigating the complex journey of Dementia caregiving.

24
Links

It's been both humbling and surprising to see the ripple effect this book has had. These conversations, interviews, and write-ups have opened doors to deeper dialogue around Dementia, caregiving, and faith. If you're curious to hear more or want to share this journey with others, here are some of the places where *My Way* has been featured.

https://www.youtube.com/watch?v=NQeDeyotIMA

https://www.rnz.co.nz/national/programmes/first-up/audio/2018821465/nz-made-sandi-wilson-s-book-my-way

https://www.youtube.com/watch?v=gLSyV_paEYI

https://alzheimers.org.nz/blogs/where-everybody-knows-your-name/

25

Man of Ivories

Sing me a song, O man
    As you tinkle those ivories of black and white
Let's sit and have a drink
A toast to all that lay behind
and all before us.
Look in my eyes and see the torment
of your bitter soul
And the ache in your heart that never goes.
O man, on ivories of black and white
Play me a tune
A melancholic dream
A nightmare of years gone by
A ballad, a lament, of years lost
Dreams forsaken, and hearts that were
smashed in your chaos.
Play me a tune, O man
Play those ivories in the bittersweet
perfection, as only you know how
And then cry

O man cry
Cry for the innocence stolen
The instruction so severe
The battles and beauty
The times of not being there
The broken dreams
The things said in anger
The bitterness
The hatred
The sweet despair
Cry for the heart that has longed for you
To hold me when my body had been so abused,
Cry for the one you lost after me
Was it pain for you to know
her sweet misery?
Cry for the marriage that went down on the way
You fulfilled your dreams
We're the ones who paid
You never come
You never are the father I dream of
O man, on ivories of black and white
Cry for all that you have lost
Look what you gained...

Sandi Reflects:

Reading this poem now, decades after it was first written, stirs a bittersweet ache in me. At the time, I penned it from a place of rawness—of unmet needs, unresolved pain, and the longing for a connection that always felt just out of reach. I hear the voice of a young woman who was desperate to be seen and held by her father, grappling with pain, disappointment, abandonment and hope all tangled together.

I had a tumultuous relationship with my father, all the way through, until I had to reconcile that he would never be what I needed, and would come to lean on me entirely, for what he needed.

The truth hurts, but after a very long walk along a beach one day, when Dad still had his right mind, we made peace.

What strikes me now is the irony—how a poem born out of longing and grief would one day sit alongside a book chronicling my dad's final years, a journey shaped by dementia. The father I once mourned in verse became the man I would walk beside through decline, caregiving, and ultimately, reconciliation.

It's okay to express your hurts and frustrations, but there needs to be acceptance in the end. For me, that acceptance came in the quiet moments—sitting beside him in the garden, holding his hand when he was too tired to speak, or laughing gently over a shared memory. These were the glimpses of grace that softened the pain and helped me let go of the expectations I once held so tightly.

About the Author

Sandi K. Wilson is a devoted child of God, a wife happily married to her fellow adventurer, a loving mother of grown children, and a proud Safta (grandmother). A passionate writer and blogger, her love of words has been a lifelong companion.

Sandi began with a blog, but it was her deeply personal books that carved her path: one about her grandfather's plight as a POW in WWII, and several stand-alone works exploring themes of faith, courage, and healing.

She is currently writing *The House of Adonai*, a visionary series of spiritual allegories, and continues to publish through her own imprint, *SKW Publishing*. Her stories invite readers into worlds marked by truth, beauty, and grace.

When she isn't writing, Sandi enjoys travelling, gardening, genealogy, and immersing herself in history and archaeology. She finds the greatest joy in spending time with her loved ones and weaving together faith, heritage, and adventure in both her life and work.

Connect with Sandi:
- **Website:** www.skwpublishing.com
- **Books:** www.sandikwilson.com

www.ingramcontent.com/pod-product-compliance
Lightning Source LLC
Chambersburg PA
CBHW071724020426
42333CB00017B/2377